MedicalCenter.com

The Key Facts on Diabetes

Everything You Need to Know About

Diabetes

I0439921

-Usable Medical Information for the Patient-

By Patrick W. Nee

www.MedicalCenter.com

Published by:

MedicalCenter.com

96 Walter Street/ Suite 200

Boston, MA 02131, USA

Tel: 617-354-7722

www.MedicalCenter.com

manager@medicalcenter.com

Table of Contents

Chapter 1: Introduction

Almost everyone knows someone who has diabetes. An estimated 23.6 million people in the United States—7.8 percent of the population—have diabetes, a serious, lifelong condition. Of those, 17.9 million have been diagnosed, and 5.7 million have not yet been diagnosed. In 2007, about 1.6 million people ages 20 or older were diagnosed with diabetes.

What is Diabetes?

Diabetes means your blood glucose, also called blood sugar, is too high. Your blood always has some glucose in it because your body needs glucose for energy to keep you going. But too much glucose in the blood isn't good for your health.

How do you get high blood glucose?

Glucose comes from the food you eat and is also made in your liver and muscles. Your blood carries the glucose to all the cells in your body. Insulin is a chemical, also called a hormone, made by the pancreas. The pancreas releases insulin into the blood. Insulin helps the glucose from food get into your cells. If your body doesn't make enough insulin, or if the insulin doesn't work the way it should, glucose can't get into your cells. It stays in your blood instead. Your blood glucose level then gets too high, causing prediabetes or diabetes.

What is prediabetes?

Prediabetes is a condition in which blood glucose levels are higher than normal but not high enough for a diagnosis of diabetes. People with prediabetes are at increased risk for developing type 2 diabetes and for heart disease and stroke. The good news is, if you have prediabetes, you can reduce your risk of getting diabetes. With modest weight loss and moderate physical activity, you can delay or prevent type 2 diabetes and even return to normal glucose levels.

What are the signs of diabetes?

- The signs of diabetes are
- being very thirsty
- urinating often
- feeling very hungry or tired
- losing weight without trying
- having sores that heal slowly
- having dry, itchy skin
- losing the feeling in your feet or having tingling in your feet
- having blurry eyesight

You may have had one or more of these signs before you found out you had diabetes. Or you may have had no signs at all. A blood test to check your glucose levels will show if you have prediabetes or diabetes.

What kind of diabetes do you have?

People can get diabetes at any age. Type 1, type 2, and gestational diabetes are the three main kinds. Type 1 diabetes, formerly called juvenile diabetes or insulin-dependent diabetes, is usually first diagnosed in children, teenagers, or young adults. With this form of diabetes, the beta cells of the pancreas no longer make insulin because the body's immune system has attacked and destroyed them. Treatment for type 1 diabetes includes taking insulin and possibly another injectable medicine, making wise food choices, being physically active, taking aspirin daily—for some—and controlling blood pressure and cholesterol.

Type 2 diabetes, formerly called adult-onset diabetes or noninsulin-dependent diabetes, is the most common form of diabetes. People can develop type 2 diabetes at any age-even during childhood. This form of diabetes usually begins with insulin resistance, a condition in which fat, muscle, and liver cells do not use insulin properly. At first, the pancreas keeps up with the added demand by producing more insulin. In time, however, it loses the ability to secrete enough insulin in response to meals. Being overweight and inactive increases the chances of developing type 2 diabetes. Treatment includes using diabetes medicines, making wise food choices, being physically active, taking aspirin daily-for some-and controlling blood pressure and cholesterol.

Some women develop gestational diabetes during the late stages of pregnancy. Although this form of diabetes usually goes away after the baby is born, a woman who has had it is more likely to develop type 2 diabetes later in life. Gestational diabetes is caused by the hormones of pregnancy or a shortage of insulin.

What are the risk factors for diabetes?

Risk factors for type 2 diabetes include older age, obesity, family history of diabetes, prior history of gestational diabetes, impaired glucose tolerance, physical inactivity, and race/ethnicity. African Americans, Hispanic/Latino Americans, American Indians, and some Asian Americans and Pacific Islanders are at particularly high risk for type 2 diabetes.

Risk factors are less well defined for type 1 diabetes than for type 2 diabetes, but autoimmune, genetic, and environmental factors are involved in developing this type of diabetes.

Gestational diabetes occurs more frequently in African Americans, Hispanic/Latino Americans, American Indians, and people with a family history of diabetes than in other groups. Obesity is also associated with higher risk. Women who have had gestational diabetes have a 35% to 60% chance of developing diabetes in the next 10–20 years.

Other specific types of diabetes, which may account for 1% to 5% of all diagnosed cases, result from specific genetic syndromes, surgery, drugs, malnutrition, infections, and other illnesses.

Why do you need to take care of your diabetes?

After many years, diabetes can lead to serious problems with your eyes, kidneys, nerves, and gums and teeth. But the most serious problem caused by diabetes is heart disease. When you have diabetes, you are more than twice as likely as people without diabetes to have heart disease or a stroke.

If you have diabetes, your risk of a heart attack is the same as someone who has already had a heart attack. Both women and men with diabetes are at risk. You may not even have the typical signs of a heart attack.

You can reduce your risk of developing heart disease by controlling your blood pressure and blood fat levels. If you smoke, talk with your doctor about quitting. Remember that every step toward your goals helps!

What is the treatment for diabetes?

Healthy eating, physical activity, and insulin injections are the basic therapies for type 1 diabetes. The amount of insulin taken must be balanced with food intake and daily activities. Blood glucose levels must be closely monitored through frequent blood glucose testing.

Healthy eating, physical activity, and blood glucose testing are the basic therapies for type 2 diabetes. In addition, many people with type 2 diabetes require oral medication, insulin, or both to control their blood glucose levels.

People with diabetes must take responsibility for their day-to-day care, and keep blood glucose levels from going too low or too high.

People with diabetes should see a health care provider who will monitor their diabetes control and help them learn to manage their diabetes. In addition, people with diabetes may see endocrinologists, who may specialize in diabetes care; ophthalmologists for eye examinations; podiatrists for routine foot care; and dietitians and diabetes educators who teach the skills needed for daily diabetes management.

What's a desirable blood glucose level?

Everyone's blood has some glucose in it. In people who don't have diabetes, the normal range is about 70 to 120. Blood glucose goes up after eating but 1 or 2 hours later returns to the normal range.

Ask your health care team when you should check your blood glucose with a meter. Talk about whether the blood glucose targets listed below are best for you. Then write in your own targets.

Blood Glucose Targets for Most People with Diabetes		
When	**Target levels**	**My target levels**
Before meals	70 to 130	_____ to _____
1 to 2 hours after the start of a meal	below 180	below _____

It may be hard to reach your target range all of the time. But the closer you get to your goal, the more you will reduce your risk of diabetes-related problems and the better you will feel. Every step helps.

Chapter 2: Diagnosis & Symptoms

How are diabetes and prediabetes diagnosed?

Blood tests are used to diagnosis diabetes and prediabetes because early in the disease type 2 diabetes may have no symptoms. All diabetes blood tests involve drawing blood at a health care provider's office or commercial facility and sending the sample to a lab for analysis. Lab analysis of blood is needed to ensure test results are accurate. Glucose measuring devices used in a health care provider's office, such as finger—stick devices, are not accurate enough for diagnosis but may be used as a quick indicator of high blood glucose.

Testing enables health care providers to find and treat diabetes before complications occur and to find and treat prediabetes, which can delay or prevent type 2 diabetes from developing.

Any one of the following tests can be used for diagnosis:*

- an A1C test, also called the hemoglobin A1c, HbA1c, or glycohemoglobin test
- a fasting plasma glucose (FPG) test
- an oral glucose tolerance test (OGTT)

*Not all tests are recommended for diagnosing all types of diabetes. See the individual test descriptions for details.

Another blood test, the random plasma glucose (RPG) test, is sometimes used to diagnose diabetes during a regular health checkup. If the RPG measures 200 micrograms per deciliter or above, and the individual also shows symptoms of diabetes, then a health care provider may diagnose diabetes.

Symptoms of diabetes include

- increased urination
- increased thirst
- unexplained weight loss

Other symptoms can include fatigue, blurred vision, increased hunger, and sores that do not heal.

Any test used to diagnose diabetes requires confirmation with a second measurement unless clear symptoms of diabetes exist.

The following table provides the blood test levels for diagnosis of diabetes for nonpregnant adults and diagnosis of prediabetes.

Blood Test Levels for Diagnosis of Diabetes and Prediabetes

	A1C (percent)	Fasting Plasma Glucose (mg/dL)	Oral Glucose Tolerance Test (mg/dL)
Diabetes	6.5 or above	126 or above	200 or above
Prediabetes	5.7 to 6.4	100 to 125	140 to 199
Normal	About 5	99 or below	139 or below

Definitions: mg = milligram, dl. = deciliter
For all three tests, within the prediabetes range, the higher the test result, the greater the risk of diabetes.

Pre-diabetes

Pre-diabetes means you have blood glucose, or blood sugar, levels that are higher than normal but not high enough to be called diabetes. Glucose comes from the foods you eat. Too much glucose in your blood can damage your body over time. If you have pre-diabetes, you are more likely to develop type 2 diabetes, heart disease, and stroke.

Most people with pre-diabetes don't have any symptoms. Your doctor can test your blood to find out if your blood glucose levels are higher than normal. If you are 45 years old or older, your doctor may recommend that you be tested for pre-diabetes, especially if you are overweight.

Losing weight - at least 5 to 10 percent of your starting weight - can prevent or delay diabetes or even reverse pre-diabetes. That's 10 to 20 pounds for someone who weighs 200 pounds. You can lose weight by cutting down on the amount of calories and fat you eat and being physically active at least 30 minutes a day. Being physically active makes your body's insulin work better. Your doctor may also prescribe medicine to help control the amount of glucose in your blood.

The A1C Test

What is the A1C test?

The A1C test is a blood test that provides information about a person's average levels of blood glucose, also called blood sugar, over the past 3 months. The A1C test is sometimes called the hemoglobin A1c, HbA1c, or glycohemoglobin test. The A1C test is the primary test used for diabetes management and diabetes research.

How does the A1C test work?

The A1C test is based on the attachment of glucose to hemoglobin, the protein in red blood cells that carries oxygen. In the body, red blood cells are constantly forming and dying, but typically they live for about 3 months. Thus, the A1C test reflects the average of a person's blood glucose levels over the past 3 months. The A1C test result is reported as a percentage. The higher the percentage, the higher a person's blood glucose levels have been. A normal A1C level is below 5.7 percent.

Can the A1C test be used to diagnose type 2 diabetes and prediabetes?

Yes. In 2009, an international expert committee recommended the A1C test as one of the tests available to help diagnose type 2 diabetes and prediabetes. Previously, only the traditional blood glucose tests were used to diagnose diabetes and prediabetes.

Because the A1C test does not require fasting and blood can be drawn for the test at any time of day, experts are hoping its convenience will allow more people to get tested—thus, decreasing the number of people with undiagnosed diabetes.

However, some medical organizations continue to recommend using blood glucose tests for diagnosis.

Why should a person be tested for diabetes?

Testing is especially important because early in the disease diabetes has no symptoms. Although no test is perfect, the A1C and blood glucose tests are the best tools available to diagnose diabetes—a serious and lifelong disease.

Testing enables health care providers to find and treat diabetes before complications occur and to find and treat prediabetes, which can delay or prevent type 2 diabetes from developing.

Has the A1C test improved?

Yes. A1C laboratory tests are now standardized. In the past, the A1C test was not recommended for diagnosis of type 2 diabetes and prediabetes because the many different types of A1C tests could give varied results. The accuracy has been improved by the National Glycohemoglobin Standardization Program (NGSP), which developed standards for the A1C tests.

The NGSP certifies that manufacturers of A1C tests provide tests that are consistent with those used in a major diabetes study. The study established current A1C goals for blood glucose control that can reduce the occurrence of diabetes complications, such as blindness and blood vessel disease.

How is the A1C test used to diagnose type 2 diabetes and prediabetes?

The A1C test can be used to diagnose type 2 diabetes and prediabetes alone or in combination with other diabetes tests. When the A1C test is used for diagnosis, the blood sample must be sent to a laboratory that uses an NGSP-certified method for analysis to ensure the results are standardized.

Blood samples analyzed in a health care provider's office, known as point-of-care (POC) tests, are not standardized for diagnosing diabetes. The following table provides the percentages that indicate diagnoses of normal, diabetes, and prediabetes according to A1C levels.

Diagnosis*	A1C Level
Normal	below 5.7 percent
Diabetes	6.5 percent or above
Prediabetes	5.7 to 6.4 percent

*Any test for diagnosis of diabetes requires confirmation with a second measurement unless there are clear symptoms of diabetes.

Having prediabetes is a risk factor for getting type 2 diabetes. People with prediabetes may be retested each year. Within the prediabetes A1C range of 5.7 to 6.4 percent, the higher the A1C, the greater the risk of diabetes. Those with prediabetes are likely to develop type 2 diabetes within 10 years, but they can take steps to prevent or delay diabetes.

Is the A1C test used during pregnancy?

The A1C test may be used at the first visit to the health care provider during pregnancy to see if women with risk factors had undiagnosed diabetes before becoming pregnant. After that, the oral glucose tolerance test (OGTT) is used to test for diabetes that develops during pregnancy—known as gestational diabetes. After delivery, women who had gestational diabetes should be tested for persistent diabetes. Blood glucose tests, rather than the A1C test, should be used for testing within 12 weeks of delivery.

Can blood glucose tests still be used for diagnosing type 2 diabetes and prediabetes?

Yes. The standard blood glucose tests used for diagnosing type 2 diabetes and prediabetes-the fasting plasma glucose (FPG) test and the OGTT—are still recommended. The random plasma glucose test, also called the casual glucose test, may be used for diagnosing diabetes when symptoms of diabetes are present. In some cases, the A1C test is used to help health care providers confirm the results of a blood glucose test.

Can the A1C test result in a different diagnosis than the blood glucose tests?

Yes. In some people, a blood glucose test may indicate a diagnosis of diabetes while an A1C test does not. The reverse can also occur—an A1C test may indicate a diagnosis of diabetes even though a blood glucose test does not. Because of these variations in test results, health care providers repeat tests before making a diagnosis.

People with differing test results may be in an early stage of the disease, where blood glucose levels have not risen high enough to show on every test. Sometimes, making simple changes in lifestyle—losing a small amount of weight and increasing physical activity—can help people in this early stage reverse diabetes or delay its onset.

Are diabetes blood test results always accurate?

All laboratory test results can vary from day to day and from test to test. Results can vary

- *within the person being tested.* A person's blood glucose levels normally move up and down depending on meals, exercise, sickness, and stress.
- *between different tests.* Each test measures blood glucose levels in a different way. For example, the FPG test measures glucose that is floating free in the blood after fasting and only shows the blood glucose level at the time of the test. Repeated blood glucose tests, such as self-monitoring several times a day with a home meter, can record the natural variations of blood glucose levels during the day. The A1C test represents the amount of glucose attached to hemoglobin, so it reflects an average of all the blood glucose levels a person may experience over 3

months. The A1C test will not show day-to-day changes.

The following chart shows how multiple blood glucose measurements over 4 days compare with an A1C measurement.

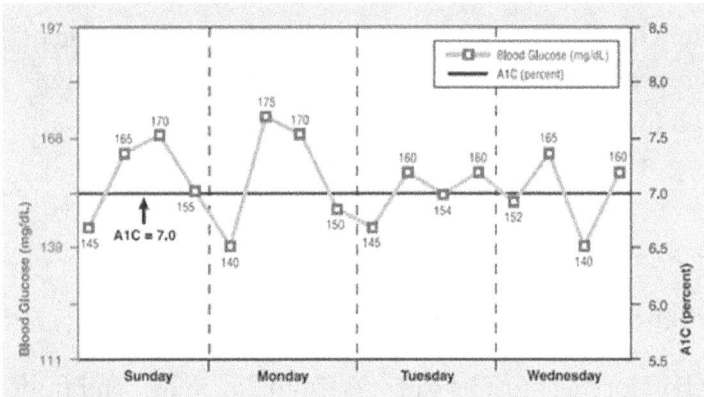

Note: Blood glucose (mg/dL) measurements were taken four times per day (fasting or pre-breakfast, pre-lunch, pre-dinner, and bedtime).

The straight black line indicates an A1C measurement of 7.0 percent. The blue line shows blood glucose test results from self-monitoring four times a day over a 4-day period.

- *within the same test.* Even when the same blood sample is repeatedly measured in the same laboratory, the results may vary due to small changes in temperature, equipment, or sample handling.

Health care providers take these variations into account when considering test results and repeat laboratory tests for confirmation. Diabetes develops over time, so even with variations in test results, health care providers can tell when overall blood glucose levels are becoming too high.

Comparing test results from different laboratories can be misleading. People should consider requesting new laboratory tests when they change health care providers, or if their health care provider's office changes the laboratory or clinic it uses for blood testing.

How accurate is the A1C test?

The A1C test result can be up to 0.5 percent higher or lower than the actual percentage. This means an A1C measured as 7.0 percent could indicate a true A1C anywhere in the range from 6.5 to 7.5 percent.

The drawing below shows the range of variation that can occur when an A1C is 7.0 percent on the lab report.

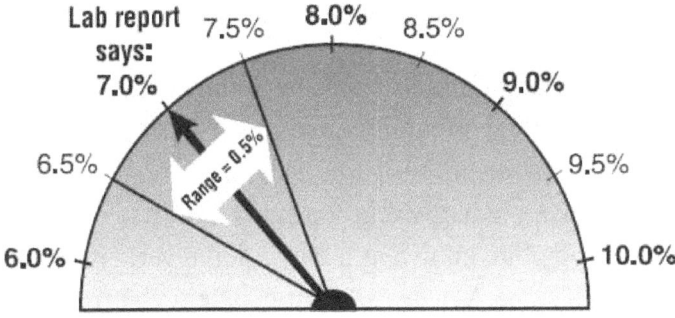

To put the A1C test into perspective, an FPG test result of 126 mg/dL could indicate a true FPG anywhere in the range from 110 to 142 mg/dL. This variation will be even greater if the blood sample is not processed promptly or is not put on ice, causing blood glucose levels in the sample to decrease. The drawing below shows the range of variation that can occur when the FPG is 126 mg/dL.

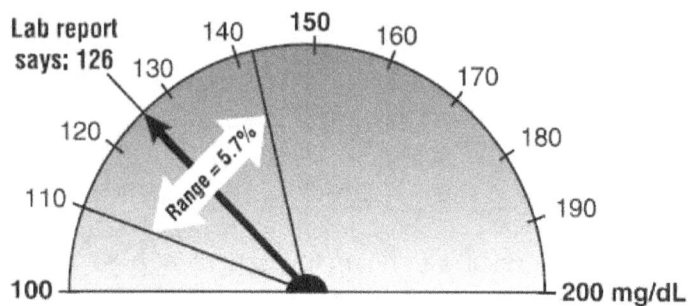

Can the A1C test give false results?

Yes, for some people. The A1C test can be unreliable for diagnosing or monitoring diabetes in people with certain conditions that are known to interfere with the results. Interference should be suspected when A1C results seem very different from the results of a blood glucose test.

People of African, Mediterranean, or Southeast Asian descent, or people with family members with sickle cell anemia or a thalassemia are particularly at risk of interference. People in these groups may have a less common type of hemoglobin, known as a hemoglobin variant, that can interfere with some A1C tests. Most people with a hemoglobin variant have no symptoms and may not know that they carry this type of hemoglobin.

Not all of the A1C tests are unreliable for people with a hemoglobin variant. People with false results from one type of A1C test may need a different type of A1C test for measuring their average blood glucose level.

False A1C results may also occur in people with other problems that affect their blood or hemoglobin. For example, a falsely low A1C result can occur in people with

- anemia
- heavy bleeding

A falsely elevated A1C result can occur in people who

- are very low in iron, for example, those with iron deficiency anemia

Other causes of false A1C results include

- kidney failure
- liver disease

How is the A1C test used after diagnosis of diabetes?

Health care providers can use the A1C test to monitor blood glucose levels in people with type 1 or type 2 diabetes. The A1C test is not used to monitor gestational diabetes.

The American Diabetes Association recommends that people with diabetes who are meeting treatment goals and have stable blood glucose levels have the A1C test twice a year. Health care providers may repeat the A1C test as often as four times a year until blood glucose levels reach recommended levels.

The A1C test helps health care providers adjust medication to reduce the risk of long-term diabetes complications. Studies have demonstrated substantial reductions in long-term complications with the lowering of A1C levels.

When the A1C test is used for monitoring blood glucose levels in a person with diabetes, the blood sample can be analyzed in a health care provider's office using a POC test to give immediate results. However, POC tests are less reliable and not as accurate as most laboratory tests.

How does the A1C relate to estimated average glucose?

Estimated average glucose (eAG) is calculated from the A1C. Some laboratories report eAG with the A1C test results. The eAG number helps people with diabetes relate their A1C to daily glucose monitoring levels. The eAG calculation converts the A1C percentage to the same units used by home glucose meters—milligrams per deciliter (mg/dL).

The eAG number will not match daily glucose readings because it is a long-term average rather than the blood glucose level at a single time, as measured with the home glucose meter. The following table shows the relationship between the A1C and the eAG.

A1C	eAG
Percent	mg/dL

6	126
7	154
8	183
9	212
10	240
11	269
12	298

What A1C target should people have?

People will have different A1C targets depending on their diabetes history and their general health. People should discuss their A1C target with their health care provider. Studies have shown that people with diabetes can reduce the risk of diabetes complications by keeping A1C levels below 7 percent.

Maintaining good blood glucose control will benefit those with new-onset diabetes for many years to come. However, an A1C level that is safe for one person may not be safe for another. For example, keeping an A1C level below 7 percent may not be safe if it leads to problems with hypoglycemia, also called low blood glucose.

Less strict blood glucose control, or an A1C between 7 and 8 percent—or even higher in some circumstances—may be appropriate in people who have

- limited life-expectancy
- long-standing diabetes and difficulty attaining a lower goal
- severe hypoglycemia
- advanced diabetes complications such as chronic kidney disease, nerve problems, or cardiovascular disease

Will the A1C test show changes in blood glucose levels?

Large changes in a person's blood glucose levels over the past month will show up in their A1C test result, but the A1C does not show sudden, temporary increases or decreases in blood glucose levels. Even though the A1C represents a long-term average, blood glucose levels within the past 30 days have a greater effect on the A1C reading than those in previous months.

Points to Remember

- The A1C test is a blood test that provides information about a person's average levels of blood glucose, also called blood sugar, over the past 3 months.
- The A1C test is based on the attachment of glucose to hemoglobin, the protein in red blood cells that carries oxygen. Thus, the A1C test reflects the average of a person's blood glucose levels over the past 3 months.
- In 2009, an international expert committee recommended the A1C test be used as one of the tests available to help diagnose type 2 diabetes and prediabetes.
- Because the A1C test does not require fasting and blood can be drawn for the test at any time of day, experts are hoping its convenience will allow more people to get tested—thus, decreasing the number of people with undiagnosed diabetes.
- In the past, the A1C test was not recommended for diagnosis of type 2 diabetes and prediabetes because the many different types of A1C tests could give varied results. The accuracy has been improved by the National Glycohemoglobin Standardization Program (NGSP), which developed standards for the A1C tests. Blood samples analyzed in a health care provider's office, known as point-of-care (POC) tests, are not standardized for use in diagnosing diabetes.
- The A1C test may be used at the first visit to the health care provider during pregnancy to see if women with risk factors had undiagnosed diabetes before becoming pregnant. After that, the oral glucose tolerance test (OGTT) is used to test for diabetes that

develops during pregnancy—known as gestational diabetes.

- The standard blood glucose tests used for diagnosing type 2 diabetes and prediabetes—the fasting plasma glucose (FPG) test and the OGTT—are still recommended. The random plasma glucose test may be used for diagnosing diabetes when symptoms of diabetes are present.

- The A1C test can be unreliable for diagnosing or monitoring diabetes in people with certain conditions that are known to interfere with the results.

- The American Diabetes Association recommends that people with diabetes who are meeting treatment goals and have stable blood glucose levels have the A1C test twice a year.

- Estimated average glucose (eAG) is calculated from the A1C to help people with diabetes relate their A1C to daily glucose monitoring levels.

- People will have different A1C targets depending on their diabetes history and their general health. People should discuss their A1C target with their health care provider.

High Blood Sugar

High blood sugar occurs when your body makes too little insulin or when your body is not able to use insulin the right way. Insulin is a hormone that helps the body use glucose (sugar) for energy. Insulin is made by the pancreas.

High blood sugar is also called high blood glucose or hyperglycemia.

Symptoms of High Blood Sugar

- Symptoms of high blood sugar can include:
- Being very thirsty
- Having blurry vision
- Having dry skin
- Feeling weak or tired
- Needing to pee a lot

You may have other, more serious symptoms if your blood sugar becomes very high.

What to Think about When Your Blood Sugar Is High

High blood sugar can harm you. If your blood sugar is high, you need to know how to bring it down. Here are some questions to ask yourself if your blood sugars are high:

Are you eating correctly?

- Are you eating too much? Have you been following your diabetes meal plan?
- Did you have a high-fat or high-fiber meal?

Are you taking your diabetes medicines correctly?

- Has your doctor changed your medicines?
- If you take insulin, have you been taking the correct dose?

- Are you afraid of having low blood sugar? Is that causing you to eat too much or take too little insulin or other diabetes medicine?
- Have you injected insulin into a scar or overused area? Have you been rotating sites?

What else has changed?

- Have you been less active than usual?
- Do you have a cold, the flu, or another illness?
- Have you had some stress?
- Have you been checking your blood sugar ?
- Have you gained weight?

Preventing High Blood Sugar

When you have diabetes, you will learn to use diet, exercise, and diabetes medicines or insulin to prevent high blood sugar levels.

You and your doctor will:

- Set a target goal for your blood sugar levels for different times during the day This helps you manage your blood sugar.
- Decide how often you need to check your blood sugar at home.

If your blood sugar is higher than your goals for 3 days and you do not know why, check your urine for ketones. Then call your doctor or nurse.

Glucose Test

A blood glucose test measures the amount of a sugar called glucose in a sample of your blood.

Glucose is a major source of energy for most cells of the body, including those in the brain. Carbohydrates (or carbs) are found in fruit, cereal, bread, pasta, and rice. They are quickly turned into glucose in your body. This raises your blood glucose level.

Hormones made in the body called insulin and glucagon help control blood glucose levels.

How the Test is Performed

A blood sample is needed.

How to Prepare for the Test

The test may be done in 2 ways:

- After you have not eaten anything for at least 8 hours (fasting)
- At any time of the day (random)

How the Test Will Feel

When the needle is inserted to draw blood, some people feel moderate pain, while others feel only a prick or stinging sensation. Afterward, there may be some throbbing.

Why the Test is Performed

Your doctor may order this test if you have signs of diabetes. However, other tests (glucose tolerance test and fasting blood glucose test) are better for diagnosing diabetes.

The blood glucose test is also used to monitor patients who have the diabetes. It may also be done if you have:

- A change in behavior
- Fainting spells
- Seizures for the first time

Normal Results

If you had a fasting blood glucose test, a level between 70 and 100 milligrams per deciliter (mg/dL) is considered normal.

If you had a random blood glucose test, normal results depend on when you last ate. Most of the time, blood glucose levels will be below 125 mg/dL.

Normal value ranges may vary slightly among different laboratories. Talk to your doctor about the meaning of your specific test results.

The examples above show the common measurements for results for these tests. Some laboratories use different measurements or may test different specimens.

What Abnormal Results Mean

If you had a fasting blood glucose test:

- A level of 100-125mg/dL means you have impaired fasting glucose, a type of prediabetes. This increases your risk for type 2 diabetes.
- A level of 126 mg/dL and higher most often means you have diabetes.

Higher-than-normal random blood glucose levels may be a sign of diabetes. In someone with diabetes, it may mean the diabetes is not well controlled. Your healthcare provider will likely order a fasting blood glucose or a glucose tolerance test, depending on your random test result.

Other medical problems may also cause higher-than-normal blood glucose levels, including:

- Overactive thyroid gland
- Pancreatic cancer
- Pancreatitis
- Rare tumors, including pheochromocytoma,acromegaly,Cushing syndrome, or glucagonoma

Lower-than-normal blood glucose levels (hypoglycemia) may be due to:

- Hypopituitarism (a pituitary gland disorder)
- Underactive thyroid gland
- Insulinoma (very rare)
- Too little food
- Too much insulin or other diabetes medications

Risks

Veins and arteries vary in size from one patient to another and from one side of the body to the other. Obtaining a blood sample from some people may be more difficult than from others.

Other risks associated with having blood drawn are slight but may include:

- Excessive bleeding
- Fainting or feeling light-headed
- Hematoma (blood accumulating under the skin)
- Infection (a slight risk any time the skin is broken)

Considerations

Many forms of severe stress (for example, trauma, stroke, heart attack, and surgery) can temporarily raise blood glucose levels.

Drugs that can increase glucose measurements include the following:

- Certain medicines to treat schizophrenia and psychosis
- Beta-blockers (such as propranolol)
- Corticosteroids (such as prednisone)
- Estrogens
- Glucagon
- Isoniazid
- Lithium
- Oral contraceptives (birth control pills)
- Phenothiazines
- Phenytoin
- Salicylates (see aspirin overdose)
- Thiazide diuretics (such as hydrochlorothiazide)
- Triamterene
- Tricyclic antidepressants

Drugs that can decrease glucose measurements include the following:

- Acetaminophen
- Alcohol
- Anabolic steroids
- Clofibrate
- Disopyramide
- Gemfibrozil
- Monoamine oxidase inhibitors (MAOIs)
- Pentamidine

Low Blood Sugar

Low blood sugar is called hypoglycemia. Blood sugar below 70 mg/dL is low. Blood sugars below this level can harm you.

If you have diabetes and are taking any of these diabetes medications, you are at risk for low blood sugar:

- Insulin
- Chlorpropamide (Diabinese), tolazamide (Tolinase), acetohexamide (Dymelor), glipizide (Glucotrol), or tolbutamide (Orinase)
- Glyburide (Micronase), glimepiride (Amaryl), and repaglinide (Prandin), and nateglinide (Starlix)

Recognizing Low Blood Sugar

Know how to tell when your blood sugar is getting low. Symptoms are:

- Weakness
- Feeling tired
- Shaking
- Sweating
- Headache
- Hunger
- Feeling nervous or anxious
- Feeling cranky
- Trouble thinking clearly
- Double or blurry vision
- Feeling uneasy
- Fast or pounding heartbeat

Sometimes your blood sugar may be too low even if you do not have symptoms. If it gets too low, you may:

- Faint
- Have a seizure
- Go into a coma

Check Your Blood Sugar Often

Talk with your doctor or nurse about when you should check your blood sugar every day. People who have low blood sugar need to check their blood sugar more often.

The most common causes of low blood sugar are:

- Taking your insulin or diabetes medicine at the wrong time

- Taking too much insulin or diabetes medicine by mistake
- Not eating enough during meals or snacks after you have taken insulin or diabetes medicine
- Skipping meals
- Waiting to eat your meals
- Exercising a lot or at a time that is unusual for you
- Drinking alcohol

Preventing Low Blood Sugar

Preventing low blood sugar is better than having to treat it.

- When you exercise, check your blood sugar levels. Make sure you have snacks with you.
- Ask your doctor or nurse if you need a bedtime snack to prevent low blood sugar overnight. Protein snacks may be best.
- Do not drink alcohol without eating food. If you do drink, have only 1 or 2 drinks at the most.

Family and friends should know how to help. They should know:

- The symptoms of low blood sugar and how to tell if you have them
- How much and what kind of food they should give you
- When to call for emergency help
- How to inject glucagon, a hormone that increases your blood sugar. Your doctor or nurse will tell you when to use this medicine.

If you have diabetes, always wear a medical alert bracelet or necklace. This way emergency medical workers will know you have diabetes.

When Your Blood Sugar Gets Low

Check your blood sugar whenever you have symptoms of low blood sugar. If your blood sugar is below 70 mg/dL, treat yourself right away. Eat something that has about 15 grams of carbohydrates. Examples are:

- 3 glucose tablets
- A 1/2 cup (4 ounces) fruit juice or regular, non-diet soda
- 5 or 6 hard candies
- 1 tablespoon sugar, plain or dissolved in water
- 1 tablespoon honey or syrup

Wait about 15 minutes before eating any more. Be careful not to eat too much. This can cause high blood sugar and weight gain.

Check your blood sugar.

If you don't feel better in 15 minutes, and your blood sugar is still low (less than 70 mg/dL), eat something with 15 grams of carbohydrate again.

You may need to eat a snack with carbohydrates and protein if:

- Your blood sugar is in a safer range (over 70 mg/dL), and
- Your next meal is more than an hour away

Ask your doctor or nurse how to manage this situation.

If these steps for raising your blood sugar do not work, call your doctor right away.

Talk to Your Doctor or Nurse

If you use insulin and you are having a lot of low blood sugars, ask your doctor or nurse if you:

- Are injecting your insulin the right way
- Need a different type of needle
- Should change how much you are taking
- Should change what kind you are taking

Do not make any changes without talking to your doctor or nurse first.

When to Call the Doctor

If signs of low blood sugar do not improve after you have eaten a snack that contains sugar:

- GET A RIDE to the emergency room, or
- Call a local emergency number (such as 911).

Do NOT drive when your blood sugar is low.

Get medical help right away for a person with diabetes or low blood sugar if they:

- Are not alert
- Cannot be awakened

Long Term Complications of Diabetes

Diabetes makes your blood sugar higher than normal. After many years, too much sugar in the blood can cause problems in your body. It can harm your eyes, kidneys, nerves, skin, heart, and blood vessels.

- You could have eye problems. You could have trouble seeing, especially at night. Light could bother your eyes. You could become blind.
- Your feet and skin can develop sores and infections. If it goes on too long, your foot or leg may need to be removed. Infection can also cause pain and itching in other areas.
- Diabetes may make it harder to control your blood pressure and cholesterol. This can lead to heart attack, stroke, and other problems. It can become harder for blood to flow to the legs and feet.
- Nerves in the body can become damaged, causing pain, tingling, and loss of feeling. Nerve damage can also make it harder for men to have an erection.
- You could have problems digesting the food you eat. You could feel weakness or have trouble going to the bathroom. Nerve damage can also make it harder for men to have an erection.
- High blood sugar and other problems can lead to kidney damage. The kidneys might not work as well and may even stop working such that you might need dialysis or a kidney transplant.

Take Control of Your Diabetes

It is important to keep your blood sugar, blood pressure, and cholesterol in a healthy range. You should learn the basic steps for managing diabetes and staying as healthy as possible. Steps include a healthy diet, exercise, and sometimes medicines. You may need to check your blood sugar daily or more often. Your doctor will also help you by ordering blood tests and other tests. All these may help you keep complications of diabetes away.

You will need to check your blood sugar level to see how you are doing.

- You will use a special device called a glucometer to test your blood sugar. Your doctor will let you know if you need to check it every day and how many times each day.
- Your doctor will also tell you what blood sugar numbers you are trying to achieve. This is called managing your blood sugar. These goals will be set for different times during the day.

To prevent heart disease and stroke, you may be asked to take medicine and change how you live:

- Your doctor may ask you to take a medicine called an ACE inhibitor or a different medicine called an ARB, for high blood pressure or kidney problems.
- Your doctor may ask you to take a medicine called a statin to keep your cholesterol down.
- Your doctor may ask you to take aspirin to prevent heart attacks. Ask your doctor if aspirin is right for you.

- Regular exercise is good for people with diabetes. Talk to your doctor first about what exercises are best for you and how much you need.
- Do not smoke. Smoking makes diabetes complications worse. If you do smoke, work with your doctor to find a way to quit.

To keep your feet healthy, you should:

- Check and care for your feet every day.
- Get a foot exam by your doctor at least every 6 - 12 months and learn whether you have nerve damage.
- Make sure you are wearing the right kinds of socks and shoes.

A nurse or dietician will teach you about good food choices to lower your blood sugar and stay healthy. Make sure you know how to put together a balanced meal with protein and fiber. Try to eat at the same times each day.

See Your Doctor Often

If you have diabetes, you should see your health care providers every 3 months. At these visits your health care provider may:

- Ask about your blood sugar level
- Check your blood pressure
- Check the feeling in your feet
- Check the skin and bones of your feet and legs
- Examine the back part of your eyes

The health care provider may also send you to the laboratory for blood and urine tests to:

- Make sure your kidneys are working well (every year)
- Make sure your cholesterol and triglyceride levels are healthy (every year)
- Check your A1C level to see how well your blood sugar is controlled (every 3 - 6 months)

Visit the dentist every 6 months. You should see your eye doctor once a year. Your health care provider may ask you to see your eye doctor more often.

Chapter 3: Treatment

Learn About Diabetes

What is diabetes?

There are three main types of diabetes:

- Type 1 diabetes – Your body does not make insulin. This is a problem because you need insulin to take the sugar (glucose) from the foods you eat and turn it into energy for your body. You need to take insulin every day to live.
- Type 2 diabetes – Your body does not make or use insulin well. You may need to take pills or insulin to help control your diabetes. Type 2 is the most common type of diabetes.
- Gestational (jest-TAY-shun-al) diabetes – Some women get this kind of diabetes when they are pregnant. Most of the time, it goes away after the baby is born. But even if it goes away, these women and their children have a greater chance of getting diabetes later in life.

You are the most important member of your health care team.

You are the one who manages your diabetes day by day. Talk to your doctor about how you can best care for your diabetes to stay healthy. Some others who can help are:

- dentist

- diabetes doctor
- diabetes educator
- dietitian
- eye doctor
- foot doctor
- friends and family
- mental health counselor
- nurse
- nurse practitioner
- pharmacist
- social worker

How to learn more about diabetes.

- Take classes to learn more about living with diabetes. To find a class, check with your health care team, hospital, or area health clinic. You can also search online.
- Join a support group — in-person or online — to get peer support with managing your diabetes.

Take diabetes seriously.

You may have heard people say they have "a touch of diabetes" or that their "sugar is a little high." These words suggest that diabetes is not a serious disease. That is not correct. Diabetes is serious, but you can learn to manage it.

People with diabetes need to make healthy food choices, stay at a healthy weight, move more every day, and take their medicine even when they feel good. It's a lot to do. It's not easy, but it's worth it!

Why take care of your diabetes?

Taking care of yourself and your diabetes can help you feel good today and in the future. When your blood sugar (glucose) is close to normal, you are likely to:

- have more energy
- be less tired and thirsty
- need to pass urine less often
- heal better
- have fewer skin or bladder infections

You will also have less chance of having health problems caused by diabetes such as:

- heart attack or stroke
- eye problems that can lead to trouble seeing or going blind
- pain, tingling, or numbness in your hands and feet, also called nerve damage
- kidney problems that can cause your kidneys to stop working
- teeth and gum problems

Know your diabetes ABCs

Talk to your health care team about how to manage your A1C, Blood pressure, and Cholesterol. This can help lower your chances of having a heart attack, stroke, or other diabetes problems. Here's what the ABCs of diabetes stand for:

A for the A1C test (A-one-C).

<u>What is it?</u>

The A1C is a blood test that measures your average blood sugar level over the past three months. It is different from the blood sugar checks you do each day.

<u>Why is it important?</u>

You need to know your blood sugar levels over time. You don't want those numbers to get too high. High levels of blood sugar can hurt your heart and blood vessels, kidneys, feet, and eyes.

<u>What is the A1C goal?</u>

The A1C goal for many people with diabetes is below 7. Ask what your goal should be.

B for Blood pressure.

<u>What is it?</u>

Blood pressure is the force of your blood against the wall of your blood vessels.

<u>Why is it important?</u>

If your blood pressure gets too high, it makes your heart work too hard. It can cause a heart attack, stroke, and kidney disease.

<u>What is the blood pressure goal?</u>

Your blood pressure goal should be below 140/80 unless your doctor helps you set a different goal.

C for Cholesterol (ko-LESS-tuh-ruhl).

<u>What is it?</u>

There are two kinds of cholesterol in your blood: LDL and HDL.

LDL or "bad" cholesterol can build up and clog your blood vessels. It can cause a heart attack or stroke.

HDL or "good" cholesterol helps remove the "bad" cholesterol from your blood vessels.

<u>What are the LDL and HDL goals for people with diabetes?</u>

Ask what your cholesterol numbers should be. If you are over 40 years of age, you may need to take a statin drug for heart health.

Learn to Live With Diabetes

It is common to feel overwhelmed, sad, or angry when you are living with diabetes. You may know the steps you should take to stay healthy, but have trouble sticking with your plan over time. This section has tips on how to cope with your diabetes, eat well, and be active.

Cope with your diabetes.

- Stress can raise your blood sugar. Learn ways to lower your stress. Try deep breathing, gardening, taking a walk, meditating, working on your hobby, or listening to your favorite music.

- Ask for help if you feel down. A mental health counselor, support group, member of the clergy, friend, or family member who will listen to your concerns may help you feel better.

Eat well.

- Make a diabetes meal plan with help from your health care team.
- Choose foods that are lower in calories, saturated fat, trans fat, sugar, and salt.
- Eat foods with more fiber, such as whole grain cereals, breads, crackers, rice, or pasta.
- Choose foods such as fruits, vegetables, whole grains, bread and cereals, and low-fat or skim milk and cheese.
- Drink water instead of juice and regular soda.
- When eating a meal, fill half of your plate with fruits and vegetables, one quarter with a lean protein, such as beans, or chicken or turkey without the skin, and one quarter with a whole grain, such as brown rice or whole wheat pasta.

Be active.

- Set a goal to be more active most days of the week. Start slow by taking 10 minute walks, 3 times a day.
- Twice a week, work to increase your muscle strength. Use stretch bands, do yoga, heavy gardening (digging and planting with tools), or try push-ups.

- Stay at a healthy weight by using your meal plan and moving more.

Know what to do every day.

- Take your medicines for diabetes and any other health problems even when you feel good. Ask your doctor if you need aspirin to prevent a heart attack or stroke. Tell your doctor if you cannot afford your medicines or if you have any side effects.
- Check your feet every day for cuts, blisters, red spots, and swelling. Call your health care team right away about any sores that do not go away.
- Brush your teeth and floss every day to keep your mouth, teeth, and gums healthy.
- Stop smoking. Ask for help to quit. Call 1-800-QUITNOW (1-800-784-8669).
- Keep track of your blood sugar. You may want to check it one or more times a day. Use the card at the back of this booklet to keep a record of your blood sugar numbers. Be sure to talk about it with your health care team.
- Check your blood pressure if your doctor advises and keep a record of it.

Talk to your health care team.

- Ask your doctor if you have any questions about your diabetes.
- Report any changes in your health.

Get Routine Care to Stay Healthy

See your health care team at least twice a year to find and treat any problems early.

At each visit, be sure you have a:

- blood pressure check
- foot check
- weight check
- review of your self-care plan

Two times each year, have an:

- A1C test. It may be checked more often if it is over 7.

Once each year, be sure you have a:

- cholesterol test
- triglyceride (try-GLISS-er-ide) test - a type of blood fat
- complete foot exam
- dental exam to check teeth and gums
- dilated eye exam to check for eye problems
- flu shot
- urine and a blood test to check for kidney problems

At least once in your lifetime, get a:

- pneumonia (nu-mo-nya) shot
- hepatitis B (HEP-uh-TY-tiss) shot

Medicare and diabetes.

If you have Medicare, check to see how your plan covers diabetes care. Medicare covers some of the costs for:

- diabetes education
- diabetes supplies
- diabetes medicine
- visits with a dietitian
- special shoes, if you need them

Tests and Checkups

You can live an active lifestyle when you take control of your diabetes care. Still, you must have regular health checkups and tests. These visits will give you a chance to:

- Ask your doctor or nurse questions.
- Learn more about diabetes.

See Your Doctor

See your diabetes doctor every 3 - 6 months. During this exam, your doctor should check your:

- Blood pressure
- Weight
- Feet

Also see your dentist every 6 months.

Eye Exams

An eye doctor should check your eyes at least once a year. See an eye doctor who takes care of people with diabetes. If you have eye problems because of diabetes, you will probably see your eye doctor more often.

Foot Exams

Your doctor should check the pulses in your feet and your reflexes at least once a year. The doctor should also look for calluses, infections, and sores.

The doctor should check every year for loss of feeling, using a special tool.

If you have had foot ulcers before, see your doctor every 3 - 6 months. It is always a good idea to ask your doctor to check your feet.

Hemoglobin A1C (HbA1C)

An HbA1C lab test shows how well you are controlling your blood sugar levels over a three-month period.

The normal level is less than 6%. Most people with diabetes should aim for an HbA1C of less than 7%. Some people have a higher target, however. Your doctor will tell you what your target should be.

Higher HbA1C numbers mean that your blood sugar is higher.

Cholesterol

A cholesterol test measures cholesterol and triglycerides in your blood. You should have the test on an empty stomach after not eating overnight.

Adults with type 2 diabetes should have this test every year. People with high cholesterol may have this test more often.

Kidney Tests

Once a year, you should have a urine test. It looks for a protein called "albumin."

You will have more of this protein in your blood if you have early kidney damage due to diabetes. But the level of this protein in urine can also be higher for other reasons.

Your doctor will also check a kidney blood test every year. This test measures how well your kidneys work.

Chapter 4: Prevention & Disease Management

Can type 2 diabetes be delayed or prevented?

Research studies have found that moderate weight loss and exercise can prevent or delay type 2 diabetes among adults at high-risk of diabetes. The results of the Diabetes Prevention Program (DPP) proved that weight loss through moderate diet changes and physical activity can delay or prevent type 2 diabetes. The DPP was a federally funded study of 3,234 people at high risk for diabetes. This study showed that a 5-to 7-percent weight loss, which for a 200-pound person would be 10 to 14 pounds, slowed development of type 2 diabetes.

People at High Risk for Diabetes

DPP study participants were overweight and had higher than normal levels of blood glucose, a condition called prediabetes. Many had family members with type 2 diabetes. Prediabetes, obesity, and a family history of diabetes are strong risk factors for type 2 diabetes. About half of the DPP participants were from minority groups with high rates of diabetes, including African Americans, Alaska Natives, American Indians, Asian Americans, Hispanics/Latinos, and Pacific Islander Americans.

DPP participants also included others at high risk for developing type 2 diabetes, such as women with a history of gestational diabetes and people age 60 and older.

Approaches to Preventing Diabetes

The DPP tested three approaches to preventing diabetes:

- <u>Making lifestyle changes</u>. People in the lifestyle change group exercised, usually by walking 5 days a week for about 30 minutes a day, and lowered their intake of fat and calories.
- <u>Taking the diabetes medicine metformin</u>. Those who took metformin also received information about physical activity and diet.
- <u>Receiving education about diabetes</u>. The third group only received information about physical activity and diet and took a placebo—a pill without medicine in it.

People in the lifestyle change group showed the best outcomes. But people who took metformin also benefited. The results showed that by losing an average of 15 pounds in the first year of the study, people in the lifestyle change group reduced their risk of developing type 2 diabetes by 58 percent over 3 years. Lifestyle change was even more effective in those age 60 and older. People in this group reduced their risk by 71 percent. But people in the metformin group also benefited, reducing their risk by 31 percent.

Lifestyle Changes

Make Healthy Food Choices

<u>Reduce Portion Sizes</u>

Portion size is the amount of food you eat, such as 1 cup of fruit or 6 ounces of meat. If you are trying to eat smaller portions, eat half a bagel instead of a whole bagel or have a 3-ounce hamburger instead of a 6-ounce hamburger. Three ounces is about the size of your fist or a deck of cards.

- Drink a large glass of water 10 minutes before your meal so you feel less hungry
- Keep meat, chicken, turkey, and fish portions to about 3 ounces
- Share one dessert
- Use teaspoons, salad forks, or child-size forks, spoons, and knives to help you take smaller bites and eat less
- Make less food look like more by serving your meal on a salad or breakfast plate
- Eat slowly. It takes 20 minutes for your stomach to send a signal to your brain that you are full
- Listen to music while you eat instead of watching TV (people tend to eat more while watching TV)

<u>Focus on Healthy Foods</u>

Find ways to make healthy food choices. This can help you manage your weight and lower your chances of getting type 2 diabetes.

Choose to eat more vegetables, fruits, and whole grains. Cut back on high-fat foods like whole milk, cheeses, and fried foods. This will help you reduce the amount of fat and calories you take in each day.

- Buy a mix of vegetables when you go food shopping
- Choose veggie toppings like spinach, broccoli, and peppers for your pizza
- Try eating foods from other countries. Many of these dishes have more vegetables, whole grains, and beans

- Buy frozen and low-salt (sodium) canned vegetables if you are on a budget. They make cost less and keep longer than fresh ones
- Serve your favorite vegetable and a salad with low-fat macaroni and cheese
- Stir fry, broil, or back with non-stick spray or low-salt broth. Cook with less oil and butter.
- Try not to snack while cooking or cleaning the kitchen
- Cook with smaller amounts of cured meats (smoked turkey and turkey bacon). They are high in salt
- Cook with a mix of spices instead of salt
- Try different recipes for baking or broiling meat, chicken, and fish
- Choose foods with little or no added sugar to reduce calories
- Choose brown rice instead of white rice
- Have a big vegetable salad with low-calorie salad dressing when eating out. Share your main dish with a friend or have the other half wrapped to go
- Make healthy choices at fast food restaurants. Try grilled chicken (with skin removed) instead of a cheeseburger
- Skip the fries and chips and choose a salad
- Order a fruit salad instead of ice cream or cake
- Find a water bottle you really like and drink from it every day
- Peel and eat an orange instead of drinking orange juice
- If you drink whole milk, try changing to 2% milk. It has less fat than whole milk. Once you get used to 2%

milk, try 1% or fat-free (skim) milk. This will help you reduce the amount of fat and calories you take in each day

- Drink water instead of juice or soda
- Eat foods made from whole grains every day, such as whole wheat bread, brown rice, oats, and whole grain corn
- Use whole grain bread for toast and sandwiches
- Keep a healthy snake with you, such as fresh fruit, a handful of nuts, and whole grain crackers
- Slow down at snack time. Eating a bag of low-fat popcorn takes longer than eating a candy bar
- Share a bowl of fruit with family and friends
- Eat a healthy snack or meal before shopping for food. Do not shop on an empty stomach
- Shop at your local farmers market for fresh, local food
- Make a list of food you need to buy before you go to the store
- Keep a written record of what you eat for a week. It can help you see when you tend to overeat or eat foods high in fat or calories
- Compare food labels on packages
- Choose foods lower in saturated fats, trans fats, cholesterol, calories, salt, and added sugars

Exercise

Exercise is an important part of managing your diabetes. It can help you lose weight, if you are overweight. It also helps prevent weight gain.

Exercise helps lower your blood sugar without medicines. It reduces your risk for heart disease and stress.

Be patient. It may take several months after you start exercising before you see changes in your health.

Talk to Your Doctor First

Your health care provider should make sure your exercise program is safe for you.

Call your doctor if you feel faint, have chest pain, or feel short of breath when you exercise.

Call your doctor if your feet feel numb or painful. Also call if you have sores or blisters on your feet.

Make sure you call your doctor if your blood sugar gets too low or too high during the day.

If you take medicines that lower your blood sugar, exercise can make your blood sugar go too low. Talk to your doctor or nurse about how to take your medicines when you exercise.

Some types of exercise can make your eyes worse if you already have diabetic eye disease. Get an eye exam before starting an exercise program. This can make sure your exercise program will be safe for you.

Getting Started

Start slowly with walking. If you are out of shape, walk for 5 - 10 minutes.

Try to set a goal of fast walking. You should do this for 30 - 45 minutes at least 5 days a week. Do more if you can. Swimming or exercise classes are also good.

Wear a bracelet or necklace that says you have diabetes. Tell coaches and exercise partners that you have diabetes. Always have fast-acting carbs with you. Carry emergency phone numbers with you.

Drink plenty of water. Do this before, during, and after exercising. Try to exercise at the same time of day, for the same amount of time, and at the same level. This will make your blood sugars easier to control.

Your Blood Sugar and Exercise

When you exercise, check your blood sugar before exercise. Also check it during exercise, if you are exercising for longer than 45 minutes.

Finally, make sure to check it right after exercise, and later on. Exercise can make your blood sugar drop up to 12 hours after you are done.

If you use insulin, ask your doctor when you should eat before you exercise. Also find out how to adjust your dose when you exercise.

Do NOT inject insulin in a part of your body that you are exercising.

Keep a snack nearby that can raise your blood sugar quickly. Examples are:

- 5 or 6 small hard candies

- 1 tablespoon sugar, plain or dissolved in water
- 1 tablespoon honey or syrup
- 3 or 4 glucose tablets
- 1/2 can regular, non-diet soda
- 1/2 cup fruit juice

Have a larger snack if you will be exercising more than usual. You can also have more frequent snacks. You may need to adjust your medicine if you are planning unusual exercise.

If exercise causes a lot of low blood sugars, talk with your doctor. You may need to lower the dose of your medicine.

Your Feet and Exercise

You might not feel pain in your feet because of your diabetes. You may not notice a sore or blister on your foot. Call your doctor for any changes on your feet. Small problems can become serious if they go untreated.

Always check your feet for any problems before and after exercise.

When you exercise wear socks that keep moisture away from your feet. Also wear comfortable, well-fitting shoes.

Fun Ways to Stay Active

Find ways to be more active each day. Try to be active for at least 30 minutes, 5 days a week. Walking is a great way to get started and you can do it almost anywhere at any time. Bike riding, swimming, and dancing are also good ways to move more.

If you are looking for a safe place to be more active, contact your local parks department or health department to ask about walking maps, community centers, and nearby parks.

- Show your kids the dances you used to do when you were their age
- Turn up the music and jam while doing household chores
- Work out with a video that shows you how to get active
- Deliver a message in person to a co-worker instead of sending an e-mail
- Take the stairs to your office. Or take the stairs as far as you can, and then take the elevator the rest of the way
- Catch up with friends during a walk instead of by phone
- March in place while you watch TV
- Choose a place to walk that is safe, such as your local mall
- Get off the bus one stop early and walk the rest of the way home or to work during the week if it is safe

Diabetes Medications

Insulin Basics

- There are different types of insulin depending on how quickly they work, when they peak, and how long they last.

- Insulin is available in different strengths; the most common is U-100.
- All insulin available in the United States is manufactured in a laboratory, but animal insulin can still be imported for personal use.

Inside the pancreas, beta cells make the hormone insulin. With each meal, beta cells release insulin to help the body use or store the blood glucose it gets from food.

In people with type 1 diabetes, the pancreas no longer makes insulin. The beta cells have been destroyed and they need insulin shots to use glucose from meals.

People with type 2 diabetes make insulin, but their bodies don't respond well to it. Some people with type 2 diabetes need diabetes pills or insulin shots to help their bodies use glucose for energy.

Insulin cannot be taken as a pill because it would be broken down during digestion just like the protein in food. It must be injected into the fat under your skin for it to get into your blood.

Types of Insulin

- Rapid-acting insulin, begins to work about 15 minutes after injection, peaks in about 1 hour, and continues to work for 2 to 4 hours. Types: Insulin glulisine (Apidra), insulin lispro (Humalog), and insulin aspart (NovoLog)
- Regular or Short-acting insulin usually reaches the bloodstream within 30 minutes after injection, peaks

anywhere from 2 to 3 hours after injection, and is effective for approximately 3 to 6 hours. Types: Humulin R, Novolin R

- Intermediate-acting insulin generally reaches the bloodstream about 2 to 4 hours after injection, peaks 4 to 12 hours later, and is effective for about 12 to 18 hours. Types: NPH (Humulin N, Novolin N)
- Long-acting insulin reaches the bloodstream several hours after injection and tends to lower glucose levels fairly evenly over a 24-hour period. Types: Insulin detemir (Levemir) and insulin glargine (Lantus)

Premixed insulin can be helpful for people who have trouble drawing up insulin out of two bottles and reading the correct directions and dosages. It is also useful for those who have poor eyesight or dexterity and is convenient for people whose diabetes has been stabilized on this combination.

Characteristics of Insulin

Insulin has 3 characteristics:

- Onset is the length of time before insulin reaches the bloodstream and begins lowering blood glucose.
- Peaktime is the time during which insulin is at maximum strength in terms of lowering blood glucose.
- Duration is how long insulin continues to lower blood glucose.

Insulin Strength

All insulins come dissolved or suspended in liquids. The standard and most commonly used strength in the United States today is U-100, which means it has 100 units of insulin per milliliter of fluid, though U-500 insulin is available for patients who are extremely insulin resistant.

U-40, which has 40 units of insulin per milliliter of fluid, has generally been phased out around the world, but it is possible that it could still be found in some places (and U-40 insulin is still used in veterinary care).

If you're traveling outside of the U.S., be certain to match your insulin strength with the correct size syringe.

Insulin Additives

All insulins have added ingredients. These prevent bacteria from growing and help maintain a neutral balance between acids and bases. In addition, intermediate and long-acting insulins also contain ingredients that prolong their actions. In some rare cases, the additives can bring on an allergic reaction.

Alternative Devices for Taking Insulin

Many people with diabetes must take insulin to manage their disease. Most people who take insulin use a needle and syringe to inject insulin just under the skin. Several other devices for taking insulin are available and new approaches are under development. No matter which approach a person uses for taking insulin, consistent monitoring of blood glucose levels is important. Good blood glucose control can prevent complications of diabetes.

- <u>Insulin pens</u> provide a convenient, easy-to-use way of injecting insulin and may be less painful than a standard needle and syringe. An insulin pen looks like a pen with a cartridge. Some of these devices use replaceable cartridges of insulin. Other pens are prefilled with insulin and are totally disposable after the insulin is injected. Insulin pen users screw a short, fine, disposable needle on the tip of the pen before an injection. Then users turn a dial to select the desired dose of insulin, inject the needle, and press a plunger on the end to deliver the insulin just under the skin. Insulin pens are less widely used in the United States than in many other countries.

- <u>External insulin pumps</u> are typically about the size of a deck of cards or cell phone, weigh about 3 ounces, and can be worn on a belt or carried in a pocket. Most pumps use a disposable plastic cartridge as an insulin reservoir. A needle and plunger are temporarily attached to the cartridge to allow the user to fill the cartridge with insulin from a vial. The user then removes the needle and plunger and loads the filled cartridge into the pump.

Disposable infusion sets are used with insulin pumps to deliver insulin to an infusion site on the body, such as the abdomen. Infusion sets include a cannula-a needle or a small, soft tube-that the user inserts into the tissue beneath the skin. Devices are available to help insert the cannula. Narrow, flexible plastic tubing carries insulin from the pump to the infusion site. On the skin's surface, an adhesive patch or dressing holds the infusion set in place until the user replaces it after a few days.

Users set the pumps to give a steady trickle or "basal" amount of insulin continuously throughout the day. Pumps can also give "bolus" doses-one-time larger doses-of insulin at meals and at times when blood glucose is too high based on the programming set by the user. Frequent blood glucose monitoring is essential to determine insulin dosages and to ensure that insulin is delivered.

- Injection ports provide an alternative to daily injections. Injection ports look like infusion sets without the long tubing. Like infusion sets, injection ports have a cannula that is inserted into the tissue beneath the skin. On the skin's surface, an adhesive patch or dressing holds the port in place. The user injects insulin through the port with a needle and syringe or an insulin pen. The port remains in place for several days and is then replaced. Use of an injection port allows a person to reduce the number of skin punctures to one every few days to apply a new port.
- Injection aids are devices that help users give injections with needles and syringes through the use of spring-loaded syringe holders or stabilizing guides. Many injection aids have a button the user pushes to inject the insulin.
- Insulin jet injectors send a fine spray of insulin into the skin at high pressure instead of using a needle to deliver the insulin.

Chapter 5: Alternative Therapies

The National Center for Complementary and Alternative Medicine (NCCAM), part of the National Institutes of Health (NIH), defines complementary and alternative medicine (CAM) as a "group of diverse medical and health care systems, practices, and products that are not generally considered to be part of conventional medicine." Complementary medicine is used with conventional medicine, whereas alternative medicine is used instead of conventional medicine.

Some people with diabetes use CAM therapies to treat diabetes. Although some of these therapies may be effective, others can be ineffective or even harmful. Patients who use CAM therapies should keep their health care providers informed

Dietary Supplements

- In general, there is not enough scientific evidence to prove that dietary supplements have substantial benefits for type 2 diabetes or its complications.
- It is very important not to replace conventional medical therapy for diabetes with an unproven CAM therapy.
- Tell your health care providers about any complementary and alternative practices you use. Give them a full picture of what you do to manage your health. This will help ensure coordinated and safe care. Medicines for diabetes and other health

conditions may need to be adjusted if a person is also using a dietary supplement.

Some people with diabetes use CAM therapies for their health condition. For example, they may try acupuncture or biofeedback to help with painful symptoms. Some use dietary supplements in efforts to improve their blood glucose control, manage symptoms, and lessen the risk of developing serious complications such as heart problems.

This section addresses what is known about a few of the many supplements used for diabetes, with a focus on some that have been studied in clinical trials, such as alpha-lipoic acid, chromium, omega-3 fatty acids, and polyphenols.

Alpha-lipoic acid (ALA, also known as lipoic acid or thioctic acid) is an antioxidant—a substance that protects against cell damage. ALA is found in certain foods, such as liver, spinach, broccoli, and potatoes. Some people with type 2 diabetes take ALA supplements in the hope of lowering blood glucose levels by improving the body's ability to use insulin; others use ALA to prevent or treat diabetic neuropathy (a nerve disorder). Supplements are marketed as tablets or capsules.

- ALA has been researched for its effect on insulin sensitivity, glucose metabolism, and diabetic neuropathy. Some studies have found benefits, but more research is needed. (There are some studies, reported from outside the United States, of ALA delivered intravenously; however, this research is outside the scope of this fact sheet.)

- Because ALA might lower blood sugar too much, people with diabetes who take it must monitor their blood sugar levels very carefully.

Chromium is an essential trace mineral—that is, the body requires small amounts of it to function properly. Some people with diabetes take chromium in an effort to improve their blood glucose control. Chromium is found in many foods, but usually only in small amounts; relatively good sources include meat, whole grain products, and some fruits, vegetables, and spices. In supplement form (capsules and tablets), it is sold as chromium picolinate, chromium chloride, and chromium nicotinate.

- Chromium supplementation has been researched for its effect on glucose control in people with diabetes. Study results have been mixed. Some researchers have found benefits, but many of the studies have not been well designed. Additional, high-quality research is needed.
- At low doses, short-term use of chromium appears to be safe for most adults. However, people with diabetes should be aware that chromium might cause blood sugar levels to go too low. High doses can cause serious side effects, including kidney problems—an issue of special concern to people with diabetes.

Omega-3 fatty acids are polyunsaturated fatty acids that come from foods such as fish, fish oil, vegetable oil (primarily canola and soybean), walnuts, and wheat germ. Omega-3 supplements are available as capsules or oils (such as fish oil). Omega-3s are important in a number of bodily functions, including the movement of calcium and other substances in and out of cells, the relaxation and contraction of muscles, blood clotting, digestion, fertility, cell division, and growth. In addition, omega-3s are thought to protect against heart disease, reduce inflammation, and lower triglyceride levels.

- Omega-3 fatty acids have been researched for their effect on controlling glucose and reducing heart disease risk in people with type 2 diabetes. Studies show that omega-3 fatty acids lower triglycerides, but do not affect blood glucose control, total cholesterol, or HDL (good) cholesterol in people with diabetes. In some studies, omega-3 fatty acids also raised LDL (bad) cholesterol. Additional research, particularly long-term studies that look specifically at heart disease in people with diabetes, is needed.
- Omega-3s appear to be safe for most adults at low-to-moderate doses. Safety questions have been raised about fish oil supplements, because some species of fish can be contaminated by substances such as mercury, pesticides, or PCBs. In high doses, fish oil can interact with certain medications, including blood thinners and drugs used for high blood pressure.

Polyphenols—antioxidants found in tea and dark chocolate, among other dietary sources—are being studied for possible effects on vascular health (including blood pressure) and on the body's ability to use insulin.

- Laboratory studies suggest that EGCG, a polyphenol found in green tea, may protect against cardiovascular disease and have a beneficial effect on insulin activity and glucose control. However, a few small clinical trials studying EGCG and green tea in people with diabetes have not shown such effects.
- No adverse effects of EGCG or green tea were discussed in these studies. Green tea is safe for most adults when used in moderate amounts. However, green tea contains caffeine, which can cause, in some people, insomnia, anxiety, or irritability, among other effects. Green tea also has small amounts of vitamin K, which can make anticoagulant drugs, such as warfarin, less effective.

Other supplements are also being studied for diabetes-related effects. For example:

- Preliminary research has explored the use of garlic for lowering blood glucose levels, but findings have not been consistent.
- Studies of the effects of magnesium supplementation on blood glucose control have had mixed results, although researchers have found that eating a diet high in magnesium may lower the risk of diabetes.

- There is not enough evidence to evaluate the effectiveness of coenzyme Q10 supplementation as a CAM therapy for diabetes; studies of its ability to affect glucose control have had conflicting findings.
- Researchers are studying whether the herb ginseng and the trace mineral vanadium might help control glucose levels.
- Some people with diabetes may also try botanicals such as prickly pear cactus, gurmar, Coccinia indica, aloe vera, fenugreek, and bitter melon to control their glucose levels. However, there is limited research on the effectiveness of these botanicals for diabetes.

Vitamin D

Vitamin D is a fat-soluble vitamin. Fat-soluble vitamins are stored in the body's fatty tissue.

Function

Vitamin D helps the body absorb calcium. Calcium and phosphate are two minerals that are essential for normal bone formation.

Throughout childhood, your body uses these minerals to produce bones. If you do not get enough calcium, or if your body does not absorb enough calcium from your diet, bone production and bone tissues may suffer.

Vitamin D deficiency can lead to osteoporosis in adults or rickets in children.

Food Sources

The body makes vitamin D when the skin is directly exposed to the sun. That is why it is often called the "sunshine" vitamin. Most people meet at least some of their vitamin D needs this way.

Very few foods naturally contain vitamin D. As a result, many foods are fortified with vitamin D. Fortified means that vitamins have been added to the food.

Vitamin D is found in the following foods:

- Dairy products
- Cheese
- Butter
- Cream
- Fortified milk (all milk in the U.S. is fortified with vitamin D)
- Fatty fish (such as tuna, salmon, and mackerel)
- Oysters
- Fortified breakfast cereals, margarine, and soy milk (check the Nutrition Fact Panel on the food label)

It can be very hard to get enough vitamin D from food sources alone. As a result, some people may need to take a vitamin D supplement. Vitamin D found in supplements and fortified foods comes in two different forms:

- D2 (ergocalciferol)
- D3 (cholecalciferol)

Side Effects

Too much vitamin D can make the intestines absorb too much calcium. This may cause high levels of calcium in the blood. High blood calcium can lead to:

- Calcium deposits in soft tissues such as the heart and lungs
- Confusion and disorientation
- Damage to the kidneys
- Kidney stones
- Nausea, vomiting, constipation, poor appetite, weakness, and weight loss

Recommendations

Ten to 15 minutes of sunshine three times weekly is enough to produce the body's requirement of vitamin D. The sun needs to shine on the skin of your face, arms, back, or legs (without sunscreen). Because exposure to sunlight is a risk for skin cancer, you should use sunscreen after a few minutes in the sun.

People who do not live in sunny places may not make enough vitamin D. Skin that is exposed to sunshine indoors through a window will not produce vitamin D. Cloudy days, shade, and having dark-colored skin also cut down on the amount of vitamin D the skin makes.

The Recommended Dietary Allowance (RDA) for vitamins reflects how much of each vitamin most people should get on a daily basis.

- The RDA for vitamins may be used as goals for each person.

- How much of each vitamin you need depends on your age and gender. Other factors, such as pregnancy and your health, are also important.

Infants (adequate intake of vitamin D)

- 0 - 6 months: 400 IU (10 micrograms (mcg) per day)
- 7 - 12 months: 400 IU (5 mcg/day)

Children

- 1 - 3 years: 600 IU (15 mcg/day)
- 4 - 8 years: 600 IU (15 mcg/day)

Older children and adults

- 9 - 70 years: 600 IU (15 mcg/day)
- Adults over 70 years: 800 IU (20 mcg/day)
- Pregnancy and breast-feeding: 600 IU (15 mcg/day)

In general, people over age 50 need higher amounts of vitamin D than younger people. Ask your health care provider which amount is best for you.

Vitamin D toxicity almost always occurs from using too many supplements.

The safe upper limit for vitamin D is:

- 1,000 to 1,500 IU/day for infants
- 2,500 to 3,000 IU/day for children 1 - 8 years
- 4,000 IU/day for children 9 years and older, adults, and pregnant and breast-feeding teens and women

One microgram of cholecalciferol (D3) is the same as 40 IU of vitamin D

Other MedicalCenter.com Publications

All Titles Can Be Found at www.Amazon.com

www.MedicalCenter.com